THE CAREGIVER'S GUIDE TO DEMENTIA

Essential Tips for Managing Dementia, Reducing Stress, and Finding Moments of Joy

Kimberly Lahr

COPYRIGHT PAGE

All rights reserved. No part of this publication may be reproduced in any form or means without prior written permission from the copyright holder.

Copyright ©2024 Kimberly Lahr

Table of Contents

Introduction 10

    How to Use This Book 14

    A Note on Compassionate Care 15

    Understanding Dementia 16

Chapter 1 17

    What is Dementia? 17

    1.1 Types of Dementia 17

    1.2 Stages of Dementia: Early, Middle, and Late Stages 20

Chapter 2 22

    Diagnosis and Early Steps 22

    2.1 Recognizing Early Signs and Seeking Diagnosis 22

    2.2 Preparing for the Journey Ahead: Adjusting Expectations 23

2.3 Finding and Engaging with Medical Professionals and Support Networks.......24

Essential Caregiving Strategies..............26

Chapter 3..27

Creating a Safe and Comfortable Environment..27

3.1 Adapting the Home for Safety and Accessibility..27

3.2 Establishing Routines to Reduce Anxiety 29

3.3 Managing Sensory Needs 30

Chapter 4..31

Communicating with Dementia Patients..31

4.1 Effective Communication Techniques for Each Stage 31

4.2 Handling Repetitive Questions and Confusion..34

4.3 Maintaining Patience and Empathy ...36

Chapter 5..37

Behavioral Challenges and Coping Strategies 37

5.1 Identifying Triggers for Agitation and Anxiety 37

5.2 Techniques for Managing Aggression and Anger 38

Chapter 6 40

Promoting Physical and Emotional Well-being 40

6.1 Nutrition and Hydration 40

6.2 Maintaining Physical Health 41

6.3 Supporting Emotional Well-being 41

6.4 Self-Care as a Core Caregiving Principle 42

Managing Caregiver Stress and Emotional Well-being 43

Chapter 7 44

Understanding Caregiver Stress and Burnout 44

7.1 Recognizing the Signs of Caregiver Stress 44

7.2 Differentiating Compassion Fatigue and Burnout 46

7.3 Addressing the Stigma of Asking for Help 46

7.4 The Importance of Self-Compassion . 47

Chapter 8 48

Building a Self-Care Routine 48

8.1 The Basics of a Healthy Lifestyle for Caregivers 48

8.2 Practicing Mindfulness and Relaxation Techniques 49

8.3 Setting Boundaries for a Balanced Life 50

Chapter 9 51

Building a Support Network 51

9.1 Family and Friends Support 51

Chapter 10 55

Coping with Guilt, Grief, and Loss 55

10.1 Recognizing and Processing Guilt....55

10.2 Navigating Grief and Loss Throughout the Caregiving Process 56

10.3 Moving Forward After Loss............. 58

Chapter 11 59

Embracing Joy and Finding Meaning in Caregiving 59

11.2 Finding Meaning and Purpose in Caregiving 60

Practical Resources and Planning for the Future... 62

Chapter 12 63

Navigating Medical and Professional Resources 63

12.1 Engaging with Healthcare Professionals... 63

12.2 In-Home and Community Resources 65

12.3 Leveraging Dementia Support Organizations.................................66

Chapter 13 68

Legal and Financial Planning for Dementia Care 68

13.1 Understanding Legal Documents for Caregiving 68

13.2 Managing Financial Affairs 69

13.3 Consulting a Legal and Financial Advisor 71

Chapter 14 72

Preparing for Future Care Transitions 72

14.1 Recognizing Signs for Increased Care Needs 72

14.2 Assessing Options for Residential Care 73

14.3 Working with Hospice and Palliative Care Providers 74

14.4 Communicating with Family and Friends about Care Transitions 75

14.5 Preparing for Emotional and Practical Aspects of Transitioning Care 75

Chapter 15 77

Future Planning for Your Own Well-Being 77

15.1 Evaluating Personal and Career Goals 77

15.2 Rebuilding Social Connections 78

15.3 Practicing Self-Care Beyond Caregiving 78

Conclusion 80

Finding Joy and Connection in the Present Moment 81

Empowering Yourself Through Knowledge and Preparation 82

Balancing Caregiving with Self-Care 83

Honoring Your Journey 83

Introduction

When someone you love begins showing signs of dementia, the experience can be a confusing and emotional journey. Caring for a person with dementia comes with profound responsibilities and unique challenges. As the disease progresses, caregivers often face an evolving set of demands that affect every aspect of daily life, from managing medical needs to coping with emotional shifts, new behaviors, and even moments of joy and connection.

This book was written to guide you through the journey of caregiving, offering practical tools and support to help you manage your role confidently and compassionately. Each chapter provides insights, strategies, and tips drawn from the experiences of caregivers and healthcare experts alike, all intended to help you navigate dementia care with greater understanding and resilience.

What You'll Find in This Guide

Caregiving for a loved one with dementia requires more than just tending to physical needs. It's a journey that involves building patience, finding empathy, and learning ways to adapt daily to new challenges. This book is organized to address each stage of the caregiving process, with a focus on practical advice and emotional support. Here's what you'll discover:

1. **A Clear Understanding of Dementia** We'll start by exploring dementia's many forms, such as Alzheimer's, Lewy body, and vascular dementia. Understanding the nature of the disease, including its symptoms and progression, can help you anticipate changes and better support your loved one.

2. **Strategies for Day-to-Day Care**
Caregiving is most challenging when handling day-to-day demands, including behavioral changes, communication issues, and safety concerns. This guide offers practical, compassionate strategies to address these challenges while fostering a stable, positive environment.

3. **Prioritizing Your Well-Being**
Caregiver burnout is a real and pressing issue. We'll look at ways to care for yourself while you care for someone else, focusing on self-care, managing stress, and finding a balance between your own needs and those of your loved one. Taking time for yourself is not only beneficial for you but also enhances the quality of care you provide.

4. **Resources for Long-Term Planning**
   Dementia caregiving often requires navigating legal, financial, and long-term care decisions. This book includes advice on future planning and connects you with valuable resources for ensuring stability and support as your loved one's needs evolve.

5. **Finding Joy and Meaning Amidst the Challenges**
   Caregiving doesn't have to be defined solely by stress or sadness. Moments of joy and connection are possible even in the face of dementia. We'll explore ways to create positive experiences, cherish meaningful interactions, and celebrate small victories.

How to Use This Book

Each part of *The Caregiver's Guide to Dementia* is designed to support you, whether you're in the early stages of caregiving or managing advanced dementia needs. You can move through the book in order, or choose sections that best suit your current circumstances. You'll find practical tips, case examples, and guided activities, all structured to provide you with insight and confidence.

Throughout the journey, remember that while you are an essential part of your loved one's care, you are not alone. Lean on the support of family, friends, and caregivers who understand the journey, and seek out professional resources as needed. You'll find that when you approach each step with compassion—for yourself and your loved one—you'll build resilience and discover moments of connection that make the journey meaningful.

A Note on Compassionate Care

This guide is rooted in the philosophy of compassionate caregiving, which emphasizes understanding and empathy in the face of dementia's challenges. Through empathy, patience, and knowledge, you can foster a caregiving experience that provides comfort, preserves dignity, and nurtures the well-being of both you and your loved one.

As you begin, remember that no caregiver is perfect, and each day will bring its own unique hurdles. This guide will offer encouragement, reassurance, and practical support as you walk this unpredictable, yet deeply human, path of caregiving.

Let's begin this journey together, one step at a time.

PART 1

Understanding Dementia

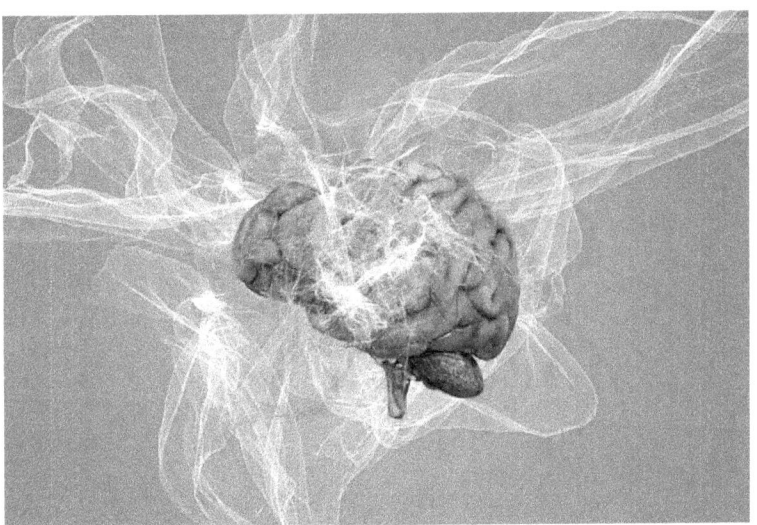

Chapter 1

What is Dementia?

1.1 Types of Dementia

- **Alzheimer's Disease**
  - **Overview**: Alzheimer's is the most common form of dementia, accounting for up to 60-80% of cases. It primarily affects memory, thinking, and behavior.
  - **Symptoms**: Early signs include difficulty remembering recent conversations, names, or events. As it progresses, patients may experience disorientation, mood changes, confusion, and behavior shifts.

- **Vascular Dementia**
  - **Overview**: Vascular dementia often occurs after a stroke or

series of strokes that impact blood flow to the brain, leading to cognitive impairment.

- **Symptoms**: Unlike Alzheimer's, which starts with memory issues, vascular dementia may present as impaired judgment or trouble with planning and organizing.

- **Lewy Body Dementia**
  - **Overview**: Characterized by the presence of abnormal protein deposits (Lewy bodies) in the brain, this form shares symptoms with both Alzheimer's and Parkinson's diseases.

  - **Symptoms**: Common symptoms include visual hallucinations, fluctuating cognitive function, and movement difficulties. Lewy Body dementia can cause rapid changes in mood and awareness.

- **Frontotemporal Dementia (FTD)**
  - **Overview**: FTD affects the frontal and temporal lobes of the brain, leading to significant changes in personality, behavior, and language skills.
  - **Symptoms**: Patients may exhibit socially inappropriate behavior, compulsive actions, and language difficulties. Memory problems usually appear later in FTD.
- **Mixed Dementia**
  - **Overview**: Some individuals show characteristics of more than one type of dementia, such as Alzheimer's and vascular dementia.
  - **Symptoms**: Mixed symptoms can make this type challenging to diagnose, as memory and

cognitive issues intertwine with symptoms like impaired judgment and mood fluctuations.

1.2 Stages of Dementia: Early, Middle, and Late Stages

- **Early (Mild) Stage**
  - **Symptoms**: Subtle memory lapses, difficulty with recent events, word-finding challenges, and slight changes in behavior.
  - **Care Focus**: Establishing routines, creating a structured environment, and preparing for gradual changes.

- **Middle (Moderate) Stage**
  - **Symptoms**: Increased confusion, difficulty with daily tasks, mood swings, personality changes, and increased need for supervision.

- **Care Focus**: More involved support, managing behavior changes, maintaining safety, and encouraging enjoyable activities that provide a sense of accomplishment.

- **Late (Severe) Stage**
  - **Symptoms**: Severe memory loss, inability to communicate effectively, physical difficulties, and increased susceptibility to infections.
  - **Care Focus**: Providing 24-hour support, ensuring comfort, managing health and safety, and focusing on quality of life.

Chapter 2

Diagnosis and Early Steps

2.1 Recognizing Early Signs and Seeking Diagnosis

- **Observing Warning Signs**: Early indicators of dementia often include difficulty remembering familiar names or places, confusion about time or events, and minor changes in mood or behavior.

- **Seeking a Professional Evaluation**: Steps for finding the right healthcare provider, such as a neurologist or geriatric specialist, for a proper diagnosis.

- **The Importance of Early Diagnosis**: Benefits include early intervention, medication options, support networks, and helping families prepare for changes.

2.2 Preparing for the Journey Ahead: Adjusting Expectations

- **Understanding the Reality of Progressive Decline**: Recognizing that dementia symptoms will evolve over time and being mentally prepared for the changes ahead.

- **Setting Goals for Both Patient and Caregiver**: Outlining short-term and long-term goals to enhance quality of life, reduce caregiver burnout, and encourage meaningful interactions.

- **Adjusting Daily Routines**: Adapting routines to align with the patient's changing needs, including setting up simplified activities, visual cues, and structured schedules.

2.3 Finding and Engaging with Medical Professionals and Support Networks

- **Choosing the Right Medical Team**: A guide to selecting doctors, therapists, and counselors who specialize in neurodegenerative conditions.

- **Developing a Communication Plan with Healthcare Providers**: Setting up a routine for regular updates, questions, and decision-making in dementia care.

- **Locating Support Networks and Caregiver Communities**: Where to find support groups, online forums, and local resources for emotional and practical support.
    - **Support for Patients**: Community programs, adult day

services, and memory care activities.

- **Support for Caregivers**: Connecting with others who understand the caregiver role, learning coping skills, and finding relief through shared experiences.

PART 2

Essential Caregiving Strategies

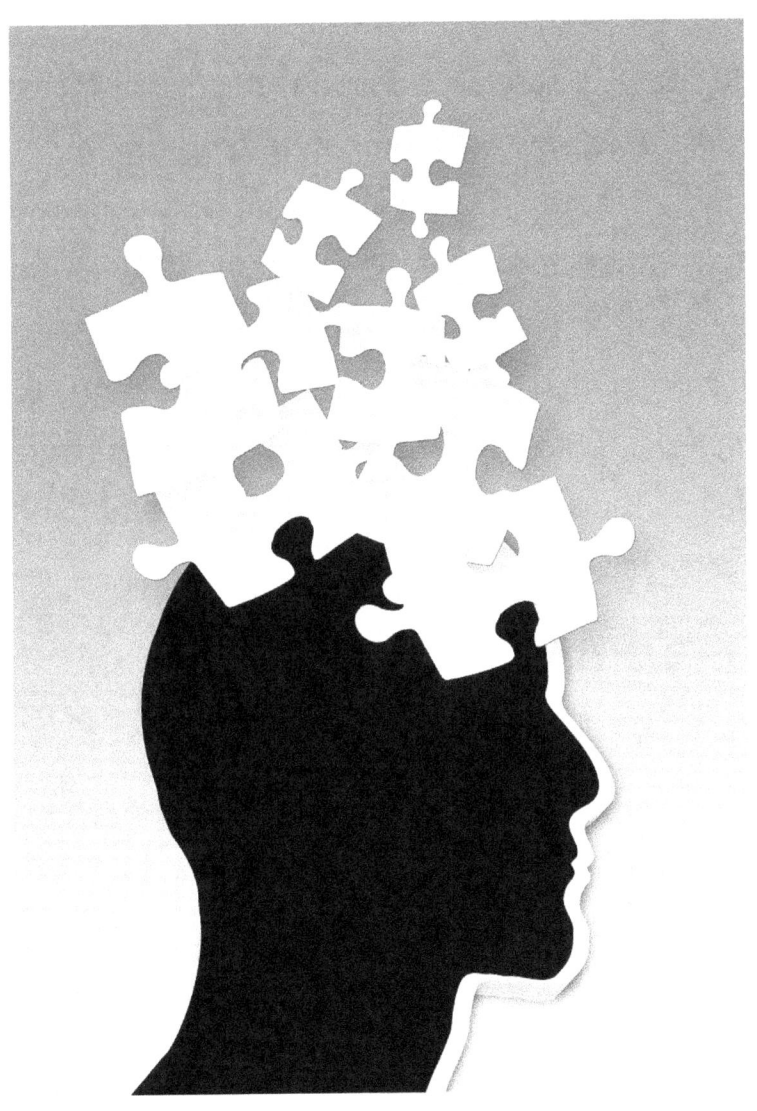

Chapter 3

Creating a Safe and Comfortable Environment

Creating a safe, comforting environment for your loved one with dementia is essential for managing their daily life, reducing anxiety, and enhancing overall well-being. Dementia can alter how individuals perceive their surroundings, so taking proactive steps to make spaces safe, familiar, and supportive helps reduce stress for both patient and caregiver.

3.1 Adapting the Home for Safety and Accessibility

- **Fall Prevention**: Dementia can affect depth perception, coordination, and balance. To prevent falls:
    - Remove rugs and clutter from pathways.

    - Install grab bars in bathrooms and near steps.
    - Ensure adequate lighting throughout the home, especially in hallways and stairways.
- **Securing Hazardous Areas**: Lock cabinets containing potentially harmful items (e.g., cleaning supplies, medications, and sharp objects). If the kitchen poses risks, consider safety knobs or locks for appliances.
- **Creating a Calm Space**: Use soft colors, familiar objects, and soothing scents. Keeping rooms uncluttered and organized can help reduce overstimulation and anxiety.

-

3.2 Establishing Routines to Reduce Anxiety

- **Why Routines Matter**: Familiar routines give dementia patients a sense of stability, control, and security. Predictability can also reduce behavioral symptoms like agitation or confusion.

- **Daily Structure**: Try to maintain consistent wake-up, meal, activity, and bedtime schedules. Make small adjustments over time if necessary.

- **Simple Visual Cues**: Label drawers or rooms to help your loved one identify where things are. This can aid in preserving some independence and reduce frustration.

3.3 Managing Sensory Needs

- **Adjusting Light and Noise Levels**: Sensory sensitivity is common in dementia. Avoid sudden loud noises, reduce background noise, and consider soft lighting, especially in the evening.

- **Utilizing Familiar Sounds and Smells**: Playing familiar music, keeping comforting scents (like lavender or vanilla), and avoiding strong, unfamiliar odors can improve mood.

- **Textural Comfort**: Use blankets, cushions, and clothing with soft textures that are familiar to your loved one, which can also offer sensory comfort and reassurance.

Chapter 4

Communicating with Dementia Patients

Communication can become a major challenge as dementia progresses. Developing compassionate communication skills can help ease frustrations and create moments of connection.

4.1 Effective Communication Techniques for Each Stage

- **Early Stage**: In this stage, patients can still communicate relatively well, though they may have trouble finding words.
    - Use clear, simple sentences and allow extra time for responses.
    - Encourage conversations by asking open-ended questions.

- Reassure them if they struggle with words; gently help them express themselves.
- **Middle Stage**: Communication becomes more challenging. Patients may become confused and lose track of conversations.
    - Focus on "yes" or "no" questions for simplicity.
    - Break tasks and information into small steps.
    - Reinforce patience and make eye contact to provide reassurance.
- **Late Stage**: In advanced stages, language abilities may diminish, and non-verbal communication becomes crucial.
    - Use facial expressions, gestures, and touch to communicate love and support.

- Speak slowly and calmly, using a soft tone.
- Engage in non-verbal activities like listening to music or looking at photos together.

4.2 Handling Repetitive Questions and Confusion

- **Responding to Repetitive Questions**: Repetition is common and often linked to anxiety or a lack of understanding.
    - Respond calmly each time, or redirect to a new topic.
    - Try to identify triggers that lead to repetitive questions.
    - Reassure them even if the question is repeated often; they may not remember having asked it.
- **Managing Confusion and Disorientation**: Individuals may become confused about time, place, or people.

- Keep large, easy-to-read clocks and calendars visible to orient them to time.
- Use reminder cues, such as labels, to help them recognize family members or understand where they are.
- In cases of acute confusion, gently remind them without arguing or trying to correct them harshly.

4.3 Maintaining Patience and Empathy

- **Understanding Their Reality**: Remember that for dementia patients, perception becomes reality. Approach each moment with empathy, acknowledging their feelings without invalidating their experience.

- **Taking Breaks When Needed**: If emotions run high, take a few moments for yourself. A brief step away can provide the patience and calmness you need to return with a fresh perspective.

Chapter 5

Behavioral Challenges and Coping Strategies

Behavioral changes in dementia can be distressing for both patient and caregiver. By understanding common behavioral challenges, you can develop strategies to manage them effectively.

5.1 Identifying Triggers for Agitation and Anxiety

- **Environmental Triggers**: Noise, clutter, and a lack of familiar cues can increase confusion and anxiety.
    - Limit distractions during conversations or activities.
    - Simplify surroundings and remove overstimulating elements.

- **Internal Triggers**: Hunger, thirst, pain, or physical discomfort can lead to agitation.

    o Observe for signs of discomfort and establish a routine that ensures basic needs are met.

    o Regular check-ins on their physical comfort can preempt many behavioral issues.

5.2 Techniques for Managing Aggression and Anger

- **De-escalation**: Speak calmly, avoid sudden movements, and give them space if they appear agitated.

- **Distraction and Redirection**: Shift focus to a calming activity, such as listening to music or looking at a photo album.

- **Reassurance**: Let them know they're safe, often repeating comforting phrases if needed.

5.3 Encouraging Positive Engagement

- **Meaningful Activities**: Focus on activities they once enjoyed, modified to match their current abilities. This might include listening to familiar music, gardening, or working on simple puzzles.

- **Daily Interaction**: Simple conversations, storytelling, and sharing familiar routines provide reassurance and engagement.

- **Recognizing Small Wins**: Praise them for small successes, like dressing themselves or remembering something familiar. These moments build confidence and create positive emotional experiences.

Chapter 6

Promoting Physical and Emotional Well-being

A person's overall well-being is crucial, especially in the face of progressive dementia. Prioritizing a balanced approach to health can help maintain dignity and quality of life.

6.1 Nutrition and Hydration

- **Encouraging Nutritious Eating**: Dementia can affect appetite and the ability to recognize hunger.
    - Prepare nutrient-rich, easy-to-eat meals and keep them on a regular schedule.
    - Offer frequent small meals and snacks, which may be easier for them to handle than full meals.

- **Hydration**: Dehydration is a common concern. Offer water regularly, or provide high-water content foods like fruit.

6.2 Maintaining Physical Health

- **Daily Physical Activity**: Gentle activities like walking, stretching, or chair exercises can support mobility and physical health.

- **Health Monitoring**: Regular doctor visits to monitor overall health, adjust medications, and catch any new issues early.

6.3 Supporting Emotional Well-being

- **Creating Moments of Joy**: Engage in activities that spark happiness, like listening to their favorite songs or sitting outdoors.

- **Validation Therapy**: Focus on validating their feelings without correcting or arguing. For example, if they feel anxious, acknowledge it and provide reassurance rather than trying to convince them they're "wrong."

6.4 Self-Care as a Core Caregiving Principle

- **Prioritizing Self-Care**: Dementia caregiving can be overwhelming, but maintaining your own health and well-being allows you to provide better care.

- **Asking for Support**: Seek respite care, ask for help from friends or family, and utilize local resources. Caregivers who take care of themselves can approach their roles with greater patience, resilience, and compassion.

PART 3

Managing Caregiver Stress and Emotional Well-being

Caring for someone with dementia is both physically demanding and emotionally complex. Caregivers often experience a range of feelings, from guilt and sadness to love and moments of joy. Maintaining your well-being is vital, not only for your sake but also to provide the best care for your loved one. This section offers practical strategies for managing stress, building resilience, and finding support.

Chapter 7

Understanding Caregiver Stress and Burnout

Caregiver stress can gradually build, sometimes without noticeable symptoms at first. Recognizing the signs of stress and burnout early is essential for ensuring your own health and continuing to provide quality care.

7.1 Recognizing the Signs of Caregiver Stress

- **Physical Signs**: Chronic fatigue, muscle tension, frequent headaches, digestive issues, and compromised immunity.

- **Emotional Signs**: Irritability, feelings of helplessness or anger, sadness, anxiety, and frustration.

- **Behavioral Signs**: Withdrawal from social interactions, neglecting personal needs, and sleep disturbances.

Over time, unmanaged stress can lead to **burnout**, a state of emotional, mental, and physical exhaustion. Burnout can reduce your patience and empathy, making it harder to provide compassionate care.

7.2 Differentiating Compassion Fatigue and Burnout

- **Burnout** occurs when caregiving demands surpass your capacity, causing exhaustion and disinterest in caregiving tasks.

- **Compassion Fatigue** involves emotional exhaustion from repeated exposure to someone else's pain, making it difficult to empathize and connect emotionally.

7.3 Addressing the Stigma of Asking for Help

- Many caregivers feel guilt or shame around needing support, as though asking for help signifies failure. Recognize that caregiving is a journey best taken with support. Seeking help doesn't mean you are neglecting your loved one; it means you value your own well-being and can care more effectively.

7.4 The Importance of Self-Compassion

- Treat yourself with the same compassion and kindness you offer others. Recognize that mistakes or difficult days are part of the caregiving experience, and practicing self-forgiveness is essential to maintaining your resilience.

Chapter 8

Building a Self-Care Routine

Self-care is essential for maintaining physical and emotional resilience in the face of caregiving demands. Building a daily or weekly self-care routine provides opportunities to recharge and reconnect with yourself.

8.1 The Basics of a Healthy Lifestyle for Caregivers

- **Nutrition**: Proper nutrition supports energy levels and mood stability. Aim to eat balanced meals, limit processed foods, and stay hydrated throughout the day.

- **Exercise**: Even short bursts of movement, like a 15-minute walk or gentle stretching, can significantly boost your mood and reduce stress.

- **Sleep**: Quality sleep is essential for mental clarity, emotional stability, and physical health. Create a calming bedtime routine to signal your body to wind down.

8.2 Practicing Mindfulness and Relaxation Techniques

- **Mindfulness Meditation**: Practicing mindfulness, even for a few minutes daily, can help you stay grounded and present. Try deep breathing exercises or guided meditation apps to promote calm.

- **Visualization**: Imagine yourself in a peaceful setting, such as a beach or forest, which can mentally reset your mood and reduce stress.

- **Progressive Muscle Relaxation (PMR)**: Tense and then release each muscle group, starting from your feet and moving upwards. This technique can help release physical tension related to stress.

8.3 Setting Boundaries for a Balanced Life

- **Protecting Personal Time**: Schedule non-caregiving time for activities you enjoy, whether reading, hobbies, or spending time with friends.

- **Communicating Needs**: Be clear and assertive about your needs with family members, friends, and healthcare professionals. Setting boundaries is vital to preventing overextension and ensuring personal time.

Chapter 9

Building a Support Network

Caregiving should not be a solitary task. Building a support network allows you to share your experiences, seek advice, and feel understood. Finding a community of fellow caregivers can make a significant difference.

9.1 Family and Friends Support

- **Asking for Practical Help**: Be specific when requesting help. Whether you need someone to sit with your loved one or handle an errand, clearly communicating these needs can make it easier for friends and family to provide support.

- **Creating a Care Team**: Designate trusted family or friends to assist with specific responsibilities, from transportation to medical appointments to organizing meals.

- **Scheduling Check-ins**: Plan regular check-ins with family members to update them on your loved one's condition and divide caregiving tasks.

9.2 Utilizing Professional Resources

- **Hiring In-Home Care**: Professional caregivers can offer respite, allowing you to rest or handle other responsibilities. Look into licensed home care agencies and review their certifications and client feedback.

- **Engaging with Respite Care Services**: Temporary respite care is available through adult day care centers, nursing facilities, or private agencies, providing caregivers with short-term relief.

- **Connecting with Dementia Specialists**: Dementia care counselors and therapists provide valuable guidance on managing specific challenges and navigating the emotional complexities of caregiving.

9.3 Joining Support Groups

- **Online Support Communities**: Many online forums, social media groups, and caregiving websites offer discussion boards for caregivers to share experiences, advice, and encouragement.

- **In-Person Support Groups**: Local hospitals, community centers, and organizations like the Alzheimer's Association often offer in-person support groups. Face-to-face interactions can provide comfort and perspective from others facing similar challenges.

- **Educational Workshops and Seminars**: Attend dementia caregiving workshops or webinars to learn new skills and coping strategies and meet other caregivers in your area.

Chapter 10

Coping with Guilt, Grief, and Loss

Caregivers often experience complex emotions, including guilt, grief, and a sense of loss. Understanding these emotions and learning to cope with them can prevent them from impacting your mental well-being.

10.1 Recognizing and Processing Guilt

- **Caregiver Guilt**: Caregivers may feel guilt for wanting personal time, making mistakes, or considering residential care for their loved one.

- **Self-Forgiveness**: Remind yourself that it's normal to have needs outside of caregiving. Self-forgiveness can alleviate guilt and help you to focus on what truly matters: providing compassionate care.

- **Setting Realistic Expectations**: Perfection is unrealistic. Aim to do your best, not be perfect. Remember that setbacks and challenges are part of the caregiving journey.

10.2 Navigating Grief and Loss Throughout the Caregiving Process

- **Anticipatory Grief**: Many caregivers experience grief as they watch their loved one decline, even though they are still alive.

    - Allow yourself to grieve the "small losses" along the way, such as the loss of memories or changes in your loved one's personality.

- **Complex Emotions and Acceptance**: Feelings of sadness, frustration, anger, and love can co-exist. Accepting these mixed emotions can reduce guilt and provide emotional clarity.

10.3 Moving Forward After Loss

- **Allowing Time to Grieve**: When caregiving ends, it's normal to feel a range of emotions, from relief to sadness to identity loss. Give yourself time to grieve the loss of both your loved one and your caregiving role.

- **Finding New Purpose and Connection**: Explore new ways to fill the time and energy once devoted to caregiving, such as joining volunteer groups, pursuing hobbies, or reconnecting with friends.

- **Seeking Professional Help if Needed**: A counselor or therapist specializing in grief can help you process complex emotions and support your journey to healing.

Chapter 11

Embracing Joy and Finding Meaning in Caregiving

Caregiving, while challenging, also offers moments of connection and joy. Recognizing and nurturing these positive moments can provide balance, relief, and a sense of purpose.

11.1 Celebrating Small Moments of Connection

- **Sharing Simple Activities**: Reading a favorite book, looking through photo albums, or listening to music together can create moments of joy and closeness.
- **Acknowledging Small Achievements**: Recognize and celebrate your loved one's accomplishments, whether

remembering your name or dressing themselves with minimal assistance.

- **Practicing Gratitude**: Maintaining a gratitude journal can help shift your focus from challenges to moments of connection and love.

11.2 Finding Meaning and Purpose in Caregiving

- **Reflecting on Your Role**: Acknowledge the significance of the care you provide. Reflect on the love and dedication you bring to your role, and recognize how you are positively impacting your loved one's quality of life.

- **Identifying Personal Growth**: Caregiving can foster patience, resilience, and empathy. Reflect on the strengths you've developed throughout the journey.

- **Connecting with Spiritual Beliefs**: Many caregivers find comfort in their spiritual beliefs, which can offer perspective and solace during difficult times. Consider prayer, meditation, or attending spiritual gatherings as a source of strength.

PART 4

Practical Resources and Planning for the Future

Caregiving for someone with dementia demands emotional strength and patience, as well as logistical planning and access to resources. Planning and knowing where to turn for support can help caregivers manage day-to-day tasks more efficiently and meet current and future needs. This section offers guidance on practical resources, legal planning, financial management, and preparing for potential transitions in care.

Chapter 12

Navigating Medical and Professional Resources

Understanding and utilizing available medical and professional resources can ease many of the caregiving burdens. This chapter provides an overview of the healthcare professionals, community resources, and supportive services that can enhance the quality of care and provide crucial support.

12.1 Engaging with Healthcare Professionals

- **Primary Care Physicians**: Primary care doctors are often the first contact for diagnosing and treating dementia. It's essential to build a relationship with a doctor who understands dementia's progression and can monitor changes.

- **Neurologists and Specialists**: Neurologists are experts in brain health and can offer insights into specific dementia symptoms, disease progression, and emerging treatments. Inquire about referrals to neurologists who specialize in dementia.

- **Geriatric Care Managers**: These professionals coordinate care, assess needs, and assist with logistical aspects of healthcare and support services. Geriatric care managers are invaluable resources for families handling multiple care needs.

- **Occupational and Physical Therapists**: Occupational therapists help dementia patients retain functional abilities in everyday tasks, while physical therapists can improve mobility and reduce the risk of falls.

- **Mental Health Professionals**: For both caregivers and patients, mental health professionals provide counseling, coping strategies, and support for dealing with grief, stress, and emotional challenges.

12.2 In-Home and Community Resources

- **Home Health Aides and Personal Care Assistants**: In-home care aides provide support with activities of daily living (ADLs) such as bathing, dressing, and meal preparation, allowing patients to remain at home longer.

- **Adult Day Programs**: Many communities offer adult day programs where dementia patients can engage in structured activities, receive meals, and socialize in a supervised setting. These programs also offer caregivers several hours of respite.

- **Memory Care Units**: Some assisted living facilities specialize in dementia care. Memory care units offer a secure environment, trained staff, and therapeutic activities to engage patients in meaningful ways.

- **Hospice and Palliative Care Services**: When a loved one reaches the late stages of dementia, hospice and palliative care can provide pain management, comfort, and emotional support to both the patient and their family. These services can be administered at home, in hospice centers, or at healthcare facilities.

12.3 Leveraging Dementia Support Organizations

- **Alzheimer's Association**: Provides a range of resources, including educational programs, support groups, and a 24/7 helpline to assist caregivers and families.

- **Local Agencies on Aging (AAAs)**: Many AAAs offer referrals to caregiver support services, home-delivered meals, transportation, and in-home services for seniors.

- **Faith-Based and Community Organizations**: Many churches, synagogues, and community groups offer volunteer support, counseling, and sometimes financial aid for families facing dementia challenges.

Chapter 13

Legal and Financial Planning for Dementia Care

Proactively handling legal and financial planning is crucial when caring for a loved one with dementia. By addressing these areas early, caregivers can help ensure their loved one's wishes are respected, their finances are managed responsibly, and potential legal issues are mitigated.

13.1 Understanding Legal Documents for Caregiving

- **Power of Attorney (POA)**: A POA authorizes someone to make legal and financial decisions on behalf of your loved one. There are different types, including durable POA, which remains effective even if your loved one becomes incapacitated.

- **Advance Healthcare Directive**: This document specifies your loved one's preferences for medical treatments, including resuscitation, life support, and comfort measures. An advance directive may also designate a healthcare proxy to make medical decisions.

- **Living Will**: A living will outlines the types of medical treatments your loved one would or would not want under specific circumstances.

- **Guardianship or Conservatorship**: In cases where an individual can no longer make decisions for themselves and no POA is in place, family members may need to petition the court for guardianship or conservatorship.

13.2 Managing Financial Affairs

- **Budgeting for Care Costs**: Dementia care can be expensive. Create a detailed budget covering current and anticipated expenses, including medical treatments, home care, respite services, and residential care if needed.

- **Long-Term Care Insurance**: If your loved one has long-term care insurance, review the policy's coverage for in-home care, nursing homes, or memory care units. This can offset some of the financial burden of dementia care.

- **Medicare, Medicaid, and Veterans Benefits**: Understand what government programs are available. Medicare offers limited coverage for dementia care, but Medicaid may cover nursing home costs for low-income individuals. Veterans' benefits may provide additional support for qualifying individuals.

- **Estate Planning**: Estate planning tools such as wills and trusts can protect your loved one's assets, facilitate the transfer of property, and designate heirs.

13.3 Consulting a Legal and Financial Advisor

- **Hiring an Elder Law Attorney**: An elder law attorney can help families navigate the complexities of dementia-related legal issues, such as eligibility for Medicaid, estate planning, and guardianship.

- **Engaging a Financial Planner**: A financial planner can guide families on managing assets, budgeting for care, and exploring benefits. Look for professionals with experience in elder care planning.

Chapter 14

Preparing for Future Care Transitions

As dementia progresses, care needs often increase. Anticipating potential transitions, such as moving to a memory care facility or transitioning to hospice care, can ease the strain and facilitate smoother adjustments.

14.1 Recognizing Signs for Increased Care Needs

- Changes in mobility, frequent falls, and increased difficulty with daily activities may signal the need for additional care.

- Escalating behavioral issues, aggression, or wandering may require a more secure and supportive environment, such as a memory care facility.

- Declining health and comfort needs may indicate a time to explore hospice or palliative care services for end-of-life support.

14.2 Assessing Options for Residential Care

- **Memory Care Facilities**: Specially designed for dementia patients, memory care facilities offer secure environments with 24/7 care, trained staff, and activities tailored to cognitive abilities.

- **Assisted Living Facilities**: Assisted living may suit those in the early stages who require help with some daily tasks but do not yet need intensive dementia care.

- **Nursing Homes**: For advanced stages, nursing homes provide comprehensive medical and personal care services.

Look for facilities with specialized dementia programs if your loved one's needs intensify.

14.3 Working with Hospice and Palliative Care Providers

- Hospice care focuses on providing comfort and emotional support for individuals with terminal illnesses, including advanced dementia. Hospice services include pain management, counseling, and caregiver support.

- Palliative care aims to improve quality of life by addressing pain, anxiety, and other symptoms, even if your loved one is not in the final stages. It can be offered in tandem with other treatments.

14.4 Communicating with Family and Friends about Care Transitions

- **Setting Expectations**: Share your loved one's condition and anticipated changes in care needs with family members. Be open about what to expect in terms of behavioral and health changes.

- **Discussing Responsibilities**: Involve family members in the decision-making process. Divide caregiving responsibilities, such as making medical appointments, handling finances, or providing direct care.

14.5 Preparing for Emotional and Practical Aspects of Transitioning Care

- Recognize that transitioning a loved one to another level of care can be emotionally challenging. Grief, guilt, and relief may coexist as you navigate these changes.

- Establish a list of personal items, photos, and familiar belongings to bring to any new care facility, which can help create a sense of home for your loved one.

Chapter 15

Future Planning for Your Own Well-Being

Many caregivers discover that caring for a loved one with dementia reshapes their own lives in profound ways. Planning for your future can help you preserve your well-being, honor your personal goals, and find a sense of purpose as you look forward.

15.1 Evaluating Personal and Career Goals

- **Setting Long-Term Personal Goals**: Reflect on goals you may have set aside during your caregiving journey. Consider making time for activities, hobbies, or career advancements you want to pursue.

- **Exploring New Paths and Opportunities**: Some former

caregivers find renewed purpose by working with dementia support organizations, advocating for caregivers, or sharing their experiences through writing or public speaking.

15.2 Rebuilding Social Connections

- Reconnect with family and friends you may have lost touch with during caregiving. Social support plays a crucial role in helping caregivers move forward.

- Attend support groups or online forums to meet others who have gone through similar journeys and can offer insight and solidarity.

15.3 Practicing Self-Care Beyond Caregiving

- Reflect on the self-care techniques you adopted during caregiving and consider integrating them into your post-caregiving life.

- Pursue activities that bring you joy and fulfillment. Whether it's travel, art, learning, or new friendships, embrace this next chapter.

Conclusion

Caring for a loved one with dementia is a profound journey that blends moments of tenderness and resilience with emotional and physical challenges. This guide has aimed to provide you, the caregiver, with a practical roadmap for navigating the various stages of dementia care—from understanding the disease itself to implementing effective caregiving strategies, managing your own well-being, and planning for the future. Each chapter was designed to equip you with essential knowledge, support, and resources so that you can embrace this journey with strength and clarity.

Reflecting on Your Role as a Caregiver

Dementia care is unique in its demands, requiring compassion, patience, and adaptability. The daily responsibilities can be both fulfilling and exhausting, and caregivers often sacrifice their own needs to prioritize those of their loved ones. Remember that you are not alone in this. Thousands of caregivers across the globe are navigating similar challenges, and support networks, professional help, and community resources are available to provide guidance and relief when needed. Embracing your role as a caregiver with compassion for both your loved one and yourself can transform the journey, infusing it with grace and resilience.

Finding Joy and Connection in the Present Moment

As you continue to provide care, focusing on the present moment can open up moments of joy and connection with your loved one. Dementia often brings unpredictability, and while this can be challenging, it can also inspire you to cherish the small, simple joys in daily life—whether it's a moment of laughter, a shared memory, or a quiet, comforting presence. Staying mindful and accepting each day as it comes can help you find peace amidst the uncertainties of the caregiving journey.

Empowering Yourself Through Knowledge and Preparation

One of the strongest tools you have as a caregiver is knowledge. By understanding the progression of dementia, you're better prepared for the challenges and changes that lie ahead. Through proactive planning and tapping into medical, financial, and legal resources, you empower yourself to make informed decisions that respect your loved one's needs and dignity while preserving your own peace of mind. Preparing for potential transitions in care can alleviate future stress and provide a clear path forward, helping you face the road ahead with confidence.

Balancing Caregiving with Self-Care

Prioritizing your own physical, emotional, and mental well-being is essential for sustaining the caregiving journey. Caregiver stress is real, and without proper self-care, burnout becomes a risk that can impact both you and your loved one. Remember to seek support, take breaks, and reach out for professional help when you need it. By investing in your own well-being, you not only strengthen yourself but also enhance the quality of care you're able to provide.

Honoring Your Journey

Caregiving is a deeply personal journey that evolves over time. Each step you take, each decision you make, and each act of kindness you offer your loved one is a testament to your dedication, courage, and compassion. Know that your efforts make a difference and that, even in the most challenging times, your commitment is both meaningful and powerful.

As you continue along this path, hold onto the insights, strategies, and resources you've gained. Lean on your support network, remember the importance of self-care, and stay open to the moments of beauty that arise even amidst the most difficult days. Caregiving may test you, but it can also offer profound growth, connection, and purpose.

www.ingramcontent.com/pod-product-compliance
Lightning Source LLC
Chambersburg PA
CBHW052336220526
45472CB00001B/442